Beauty Unveiled

Collagen Supplements, Diet, and the Secret to Radiant Skin

PUBLISHED BY: Ditya Zulkarnain

Table of Contents

Introduction

Welcome to "Beauty Unveiled: Collagen Supplements, Diet, and the Secret to Radiant Skin". In this book, we embark on a journey to uncover the powerful relationship between collagen, dietary supplements, and achieving glowing, youthful skin.

In today's world, where skincare trends come and go, and beauty routines become increasingly complex, one fundamental truth remains: healthy, radiant skin begins from within. Collagen, a vital protein found abundantly in our bodies, plays a pivotal role in maintaining skin elasticity, firmness, and overall youthful appearance.

Through the pages of this book, we will delve into the science behind collagen, exploring how it works within our bodies and its specific benefits for skin health. We'll discuss different types of collagen supplements and how to choose the right one for your needs, backed by scientific research and expert insights.

But beauty isn't just about what you put on your skin—it's also deeply influenced by what you put into your body. Our dietary choices can significantly impact the health and appearance of our skin. We'll explore the essential nutrients that support collagen production and how to incorporate them into a balanced diet for optimal skin health.

Moreover, "Beauty Unveiled" isn't just about theory; it's a practical guide. You'll discover actionable tips on integrating collagen supplements into your daily routine, creating DIY skincare treatments, and adopting lifestyle habits that promote radiant skin from the inside out.

Whether you're just beginning to explore the world of skincare or seeking to enhance your existing regimen, this book is your comprehensive companion to achieving and maintaining beautiful, glowing skin naturally. Let's uncover the secrets to unlocking your skin's potential and embracing a more confident, radiant you.

Understanding Collagen

What is Collagen?

Collagen is often referred to as the "glue" that holds the body together, and for good reason—it's the most abundant protein in our bodies, serving as a foundational building block for skin, bones, muscles, tendons, and ligaments. In the context of skincare and beauty, collagen plays a crucial role in maintaining the elasticity, firmness, and overall youthful appearance of our skin.

The Structure and Function of Collagen

Structurally, collagen is a fibrous protein that forms long chains of amino acids twisted together like a triple helix. This unique structure provides strength and support to various tissues throughout the body. There are several types of collagen, each with specific functions and distributions in different parts of the body. However, when it comes to skin health, the most abundant types are Type I, Type II, and Type III collagen.

Collagen and Skin Health

In the skin, collagen fibers are responsible for maintaining its structure and resilience. They provide the framework that supports the outer layer (epidermis) and the underlying dermis. As we age, the production of collagen naturally declines, leading to common signs of aging such as wrinkles, sagging skin, and loss of elasticity.

The Role of Collagen Supplements

Recognizing the vital role collagen plays in skin health, many people turn to collagen supplements as a way to support and enhance their body's natural collagen production. Collagen supplements come in various forms, including powders, capsules, and drinks, typically derived from animal sources such as bovine (cow), porcine (pig), or marine (fish) collagen.

Benefits of Collagen Supplements for Skin

Research suggests that collagen supplements can help improve skin elasticity, hydration, and overall appearance. By providing amino acids such as glycine, proline, and hydroxyproline—essential for collagen synthesis—these supplements support the body's ability to rebuild and repair skin tissues.

Choosing the Right Collagen Supplement

When selecting a collagen supplement, it's essential to consider factors such as the type of collagen used, its bioavailability (how easily it is absorbed by the body), and any additional ingredients that may enhance its effectiveness. Consulting with a healthcare provider or dermatologist can also provide valuable guidance based on individual health needs and goals.

Integrating Collagen into Your Beauty Routine

In addition to supplements, collagen can be incorporated into skincare products such as creams, serums, and masks. These topical treatments aim to deliver collagen directly to the skin, helping to improve moisture retention, reduce fine lines, and promote a smoother complexion.

Importance of Collagen for Skin Health

Collagen is not just a buzzword in the world of skincare; it's a fundamental protein that plays a crucial role in maintaining the health, elasticity, and youthful appearance of our skin. Understanding its significance can illuminate why collagen is often touted as a cornerstone of effective skincare routines.

Structural Integrity and Support

At its core, collagen serves as the structural framework for our skin. It forms a network of fibers that provide strength, stability, and firmness to the skin's structure. This framework is essential for maintaining the integrity of the skin's layers, including the epidermis (outer layer) and the dermis (underlying layer).

Maintaining Skin Elasticity

One of the hallmarks of youthful skin is its elasticity—the ability to stretch and bounce back. Collagen fibers contribute significantly to this elasticity by allowing the skin to withstand stretching forces without losing its shape. As we age and collagen production naturally declines, the skin may start to sag and develop fine lines and wrinkles due to reduced elasticity.

Hydration and Moisture Retention

Collagen also plays a role in maintaining skin hydration. It works in conjunction with another protein called elastin to support the skin's ability to retain moisture. This hydration is crucial for maintaining a smooth, plump appearance and reducing the visibility of wrinkles and lines.

Supporting Wound Healing and Repair

Beyond its structural role, collagen is involved in the skin's natural healing processes. When the skin is injured or damaged, collagen helps to rebuild and repair the tissues, promoting faster healing and minimizing scarring. This regenerative capacity underscores collagen's importance not only in daily skincare but also in recovering from injuries or surgeries.

Natural Aging and Collagen Decline

As we age, our body's ability to produce collagen naturally declines. Factors such as sun exposure, pollution, smoking, and poor nutrition can accelerate this decline. The result is visible signs of aging, including wrinkles, sagging skin, and a loss of overall skin firmness. By understanding how collagen contributes to skin health, we can better appreciate the importance of replenishing and supporting its production.

The Role of Collagen Supplements and Skincare Products

Given its critical role in skin health, many individuals turn to collagen supplements and skincare products formulated with collagen. These supplements aim to provide the body with the building blocks necessary for collagen synthesis, such as amino acids like glycine, proline, and hydroxyproline. Additionally, topical skincare products containing collagen or collagen-boosting ingredients can help nourish the skin externally, supporting its structure and appearance.

Types of Collagen Supplements

Collagen supplements have gained popularity for their potential to support skin health, promote joint function, and aid in overall wellness. Understanding the different types of collagen supplements available can help you choose the most suitable option for your specific needs and goals. In "Beauty Unveiled: Collagen Supplements, Diet, and the Secret to Radiant Skin", we explore the various types of collagen supplements and their benefits.

1. Type I Collagen

Type I collagen is the most abundant type of collagen in the body and is primarily found in the skin, bones, tendons, and ligaments. It provides structure and strength to these tissues, contributing to skin elasticity and firmness. Type I collagen supplements are often derived from bovine (cow) or marine (fish) sources. They are widely used to support skin hydration, reduce wrinkles, and improve overall skin texture.

2. Type II Collagen

Type II collagen is mainly present in cartilage, which is essential for joint health and mobility. It helps maintain the integrity and cushioning properties of cartilage, making it beneficial for individuals experiencing joint discomfort or looking to support joint function. Type II collagen supplements are commonly sourced from chicken sternum or other avian sources.

3. Type III Collagen

Type III collagen is found alongside Type I collagen and is crucial for maintaining the structure and elasticity of tissues such as skin, muscles, and blood vessels. It supports skin firmness and resilience, often complementing Type I collagen in skin health supplements. Like Type I collagen, Type III collagen supplements are typically derived from bovine or marine sources.

4. Multi-Collagen Blends

Multi-collagen supplements contain a combination of different types of collagen, such as Type I, Type II, Type III, and sometimes Type V and Type X. These blends aim to provide comprehensive support for various aspects of skin, joint, and overall body health. By incorporating multiple types of collagen, these supplements offer a more holistic approach to supporting collagen production throughout the body.

Choosing the Right Collagen Supplement

When selecting a collagen supplement, consider factors such as its source, bioavailability (how easily it is absorbed by the body), additional ingredients, and potential allergens. Bovine collagen is typically rich in Type I and Type III collagen, while marine collagen often provides Type I collagen with smaller peptides that may be more easily absorbed.

Incorporating Collagen into Your Beauty Routine

Whether you choose a specific type of collagen supplement or opt for a multi-collagen blend, incorporating collagen into your daily routine can help support skin elasticity, hydration, and overall radiance. Additionally, topical skincare products containing collagen or collagen-boosting ingredients can complement your supplement regimen, enhancing external nourishment and support for your skin.

The Science Behind Collagen Supplements

How Collagen Works in the Body

Collagen is often hailed as the cornerstone of healthy, youthful skin, but its benefits extend far beyond just skincare. Understanding how collagen works in the body can illuminate its critical role in maintaining overall health and well-being. In "Beauty Unveiled: Collagen Supplements, Diet, and the Secret to Radiant Skin", we delve into the mechanisms through which collagen supports various bodily functions.

Structural Support

At its essence, collagen is a fibrous protein that forms a framework or scaffold for tissues throughout the body. It provides structural support and strength to the skin, bones, muscles, tendons, ligaments, and other connective tissues. This structural integrity is crucial for maintaining the shape and function of these tissues, contributing to overall mobility, flexibility, and stability.

Skin Health and Elasticity

In the skin, collagen fibers form a dense network within the dermis, the deeper layer of skin beneath the epidermis. This network supports the epidermis and gives the skin its firm, smooth appearance. Collagen also plays a key role in skin elasticity—the ability of the skin to stretch and recoil without losing its shape. As we age, collagen production naturally declines, leading to visible signs of aging such as wrinkles, sagging skin, and loss of elasticity.

Joint Function and Mobility

Collagen is a major component of cartilage, the flexible tissue that cushions joints and allows for smooth movement. In joints, collagen helps maintain the integrity and resilience of cartilage, which is essential for reducing friction between bones and supporting joint flexibility and mobility. Supplementing with collagen may help support joint health, alleviate discomfort, and promote overall joint function, especially in individuals experiencing age-related joint issues.

Muscle and Bone Strength

Collagen also contributes to muscle and bone health. It provides structural support to muscles, aiding in muscle contraction and movement. In bones, collagen works alongside minerals like calcium and phosphorus to form a strong, resilient framework that supports bone density and strength. Maintaining adequate collagen levels is crucial for preserving bone mass and reducing the risk of fractures and osteoporosis.

Collagen Synthesis and Production

The body naturally produces collagen through a complex process that involves various enzymes, amino acids, and cofactors. Essential amino acids such as glycine, proline, and hydroxyproline are particularly important for collagen synthesis. Vitamin C is also critical as it helps facilitate collagen production by supporting the enzymes involved in collagen synthesis.

Impact of Lifestyle Factors

Several lifestyle factors can influence collagen production and degradation. Factors such as UV exposure, smoking, poor nutrition, and chronic stress can accelerate collagen breakdown and contribute to premature aging of the skin and joints. Adopting a healthy lifestyle that includes a balanced diet, regular exercise, adequate hydration, and sun protection can help support collagen synthesis and maintain optimal collagen levels in the body.

Benefits of Collagen Supplements

Collagen supplements have garnered attention in recent years for their potential to enhance skin health, support joint function, and promote overall well-being. In "Beauty Unveiled: Collagen Supplements, Diet, and the Secret to Radiant Skin", we explore the proven benefits of incorporating collagen supplements into your daily routine.

1. Improved Skin Elasticity and Hydration

One of the primary reasons people turn to collagen supplements is their ability to improve skin elasticity and hydration. Collagen plays a crucial role in maintaining the structure of the skin's dermal layer, where it supports the firmness and resilience that contribute to a youthful appearance. Supplementing with collagen peptides or hydrolyzed collagen has been shown to increase skin hydration levels, reduce dryness, and enhance elasticity, thereby diminishing the appearance of fine lines and wrinkles.

2. Reduction in Wrinkle Depth and Appearance

As we age, the natural production of collagen in the body decreases, leading to the formation of wrinkles and lines on the skin. Collagen supplements can help counteract this decline by providing the necessary building blocks—such as amino acids like glycine, proline, and hydroxyproline—to support collagen synthesis. Studies have indicated that regular intake of collagen supplements may lead to a reduction in wrinkle depth and overall improvement in skin texture and smoothness.

3. Support for Joint Health and Mobility

Collagen is a crucial component of cartilage, the flexible tissue that cushions joints and facilitates smooth movement. Supplementing with collagen peptides or Type II collagen supplements has been shown to support joint health by promoting the regeneration of cartilage tissue and reducing joint discomfort. This can be particularly beneficial for individuals with osteoarthritis or those experiencing age-related joint issues.

4. Stronger Hair and Nails

Collagen supplements can also contribute to the strength and health of hair and nails. Collagen is a key protein in the structure of hair follicles and nail beds, helping to maintain their strength and integrity. By supporting collagen production through supplementation, individuals may experience thicker hair, reduced brittleness, and improved nail growth.

5. Gut Health and Digestive Support

Beyond its benefits for skin and joints, collagen plays a role in supporting gut health. Collagen contains amino acids that help maintain the integrity of the intestinal lining and support digestive function. This can aid in reducing symptoms of leaky gut syndrome and promoting overall digestive wellness.

6. Muscle Mass and Metabolism Support

Collagen peptides have been studied for their potential to support muscle mass and metabolism. As a protein-rich supplement, collagen peptides can contribute to muscle repair and growth, especially when combined with resistance training. Additionally, collagen peptides may support healthy metabolism by increasing lean muscle mass and enhancing energy expenditure.

Choosing the Right Collagen Supplement

When selecting a collagen supplement, consider factors such as its source (bovine, marine, or chicken), bioavailability (how well it is absorbed by the body), additional ingredients, and any potential allergens. It's essential to consult with a healthcare provider or dermatologist to determine the most appropriate type and dosage of collagen supplement based on your individual health needs and goals.

Choosing the Right Collagen Supplement

Selecting the right collagen supplement is crucial to optimizing its benefits for skin health, joint support, and overall well-being. With various types and formulations available on the market, understanding key factors can help you make an informed decision tailored to your specific needs. In "Beauty Unveiled: Collagen Supplements, Diet, and the Secret to Radiant Skin", we explore how to choose the right collagen supplement effectively.

1. Type of Collagen

Collagen supplements typically come from different sources, each containing specific types of collagen. The most common types used in supplements include Type I, Type II, and Type III collagen:

- **Type I collagen** is abundant in skin, bones, tendons, and ligaments, supporting skin elasticity and structure.
- **Type II collagen** is predominant in cartilage, benefiting joint health and mobility.
- **Type III collagen** works alongside Type I collagen in skin and blood vessels, contributing to skin firmness and elasticity.

Depending on your health goals, you may choose a single-type collagen supplement or a multi-collagen blend that combines several types for comprehensive benefits.

2. Source of Collagen

Collagen supplements are derived from various sources, including:

- **Bovine collagen:** Extracted from cows, it is rich in Type I and Type III collagen.
- **Marine collagen:** Derived from fish sources, it typically contains Type I collagen with smaller peptides that may be more easily absorbed.
- **Chicken collagen:** Often used for Type II collagen supplements, beneficial for joint health.

Consider your dietary preferences, potential allergies, and the bioavailability of the collagen source when selecting the right supplement.

3. Bioavailability and Absorption

The bioavailability of collagen supplements refers to how well the body can absorb and utilize the collagen peptides. Factors influencing bioavailability include the molecular weight of collagen peptides and the presence of additional ingredients that enhance absorption, such as vitamin C or digestive enzymes. Look for supplements with hydrolyzed collagen, where collagen molecules are broken down into smaller peptides for better absorption.

4. Additional Ingredients

Collagen supplements may contain additional ingredients aimed at enhancing their efficacy or providing complementary benefits:

- **Vitamin C:** Essential for collagen synthesis and skin health.
- **Hyaluronic acid:** Supports hydration and skin elasticity.
- **Antioxidants:** Protect against oxidative stress and promote skin rejuvenation.

Check the ingredient list to ensure it aligns with your goals and dietary preferences, and be mindful of any additives or allergens that may be present.

5. Quality and Purity

Opt for collagen supplements from reputable brands that prioritize quality and purity. Look for certifications or third-party testing that verifies the product's potency, purity, and absence of contaminants. Choose supplements that are free from unnecessary fillers, artificial ingredients, or allergens that may compromise your health or skin.

6. Consultation with Healthcare Provider

Before starting any new supplement regimen, especially if you have underlying health conditions or concerns, consult with a healthcare provider or dermatologist. They can offer personalized advice based on your individual health status, potential interactions with medications, and specific goals for skin health and overall well-being.

Dietary Foundations for Radiant Skin

Nutrients Essential for Skin Health

Achieving radiant, youthful skin goes beyond skincare products and treatments—it begins with nourishing your body from within. In "Beauty Unveiled: Collagen Supplements, Diet, and the Secret to Radiant Skin", we explore the essential nutrients that play a crucial role in supporting skin health and enhancing your natural beauty.

1. Vitamin C

Vitamin C is a powerful antioxidant that plays a pivotal role in collagen synthesis. Collagen is essential for maintaining skin elasticity, firmness, and overall structure. Vitamin C supports this process by aiding in the production of collagen fibers and protecting existing collagen from damage caused by free radicals. Incorporating vitamin C-rich foods such as citrus fruits, berries, bell peppers, and leafy greens into your diet can promote skin hydration, reduce wrinkles, and improve skin texture.

2. Vitamin E

Another potent antioxidant, vitamin E helps protect the skin from oxidative stress and damage caused by UV rays and environmental pollutants. It works synergistically with vitamin C to neutralize free radicals and support collagen production. Vitamin E also assists in maintaining skin elasticity and moisture levels, contributing to a smoother, more youthful complexion. Sources of vitamin E include nuts, seeds, spinach, and vegetable oils.

3. Omega-3 Fatty Acids

Omega-3 fatty acids are essential fats that are crucial for maintaining healthy cell membranes, including those of the skin. They support skin barrier function, helping to lock in moisture and keep irritants out. Omega-3s also have anti-inflammatory properties, which can reduce redness, inflammation, and signs of acne or eczema. Fatty fish such as salmon, mackerel, and sardines, as well as flaxseeds, chia seeds, and walnuts, are excellent sources of omega-3 fatty acids.

4. B Vitamins

Several B vitamins contribute to skin health by supporting various aspects of skin function and repair:

- **Biotin (B7):** Known as the "beauty vitamin," biotin promotes healthy hair, skin, and nails. It helps maintain skin moisture levels and supports the production of fatty acids essential for skin health. Biotin-rich foods include eggs, nuts, whole grains, and avocado.
- **Niacin (B3):** Niacin improves skin barrier function and enhances the appearance of aging skin by reducing fine lines, wrinkles, and hyperpigmentation. It also boosts circulation to the skin, promoting a healthy glow. Foods rich in niacin include meat, fish, peanuts, and mushrooms.
- **Riboflavin (B2) and Pantothenic Acid (B5):** These B vitamins contribute to skin repair and maintenance, supporting the regeneration of skin cells and promoting a clear complexion. They can be found in dairy products, whole grains, lean meats, and legumes.

5. Zinc

Zinc is an essential mineral that plays a crucial role in skin health and healing. It helps regulate oil production, reduces inflammation, and supports the immune system's response to infections or wounds. Zinc deficiency can contribute to skin conditions such as acne or eczema. Incorporate zinc-rich foods such as oysters, red meat, poultry, beans, and nuts into your diet to support healthy skin function.

6. Antioxidants

In addition to vitamins C and E, other antioxidants such as selenium, beta-carotene, and flavonoids are vital for protecting the skin from oxidative damage. They neutralize free radicals generated by UV exposure, pollution, and stress, helping to prevent premature aging and maintain skin health. Include a variety of colorful fruits and vegetables, green tea, and dark chocolate in your diet to benefit from a wide range of antioxidants.

Foods Rich in Collagen-Boosting Nutrients

Achieving radiant, youthful skin involves more than just skincare products—it begins with nourishing your body with essential nutrients that support collagen production and skin health. In "Beauty Unveiled: Collagen Supplements, Diet, and the Secret to Radiant Skin", we explore a variety of foods rich in collagen-boosting nutrients to help you enhance your natural beauty from the inside out.

1. Bone Broth

Bone broth is a nutrient-dense food rich in collagen, minerals, and amino acids that support skin elasticity and joint health. When bones simmer in water for an extended period, collagen from the bones breaks down into gelatin and essential amino acids such as glycine, proline, and hydroxyproline. Regular consumption of bone broth can provide these building blocks for collagen synthesis and promote healthy, glowing skin.

2. Fish and Seafood

Fish and seafood, particularly those with edible bones and skin, are excellent sources of collagen-boosting nutrients like Type I collagen peptides and omega-3 fatty acids. Marine collagen derived from fish contains peptides that are easily absorbed and utilized by the body to support skin elasticity and hydration. Include fatty fish such as salmon, mackerel, and sardines in your diet to benefit from their collagen-rich properties and omega-3 content.

3. Eggs

Eggs are a versatile and nutrient-dense food that contains essential amino acids, including proline and lysine, which are important for collagen production. The egg white, in particular, is rich in proline, while the yolk provides biotin, a B vitamin essential for healthy skin, hair, and nails. Incorporate eggs into your diet to support collagen synthesis and promote overall skin health.

4. Citrus Fruits

Citrus fruits such as oranges, grapefruits, lemons, and limes are abundant sources of vitamin C, a critical nutrient for collagen synthesis. Vitamin C plays a key role in converting proline and lysine into collagen fibers and protecting collagen from oxidative damage caused by free radicals. Regular consumption of citrus fruits can help maintain skin elasticity, reduce wrinkles, and promote a brighter complexion.

5. Berries

Berries such as strawberries, blueberries, raspberries, and blackberries are packed with antioxidants, including vitamin C and flavonoids, which support collagen production and protect the skin from environmental stressors. These antioxidants neutralize free radicals that can damage collagen and contribute to premature aging. Enjoy a variety of berries as a snack, in smoothies, or added to yogurt for their collagen-boosting benefits.

6. Leafy Greens

Leafy greens like spinach, kale, Swiss chard, and collard greens are rich in vitamins C and E, as well as beta-carotene and other antioxidants that promote collagen synthesis and protect skin cells from damage. These nutrient-dense greens also provide minerals such as magnesium and zinc, which are essential for skin health and regeneration. Incorporate leafy greens into salads, soups, or smoothies to support your skin's natural radiance.

7. Nuts and Seeds

Nuts and seeds such as almonds, walnuts, chia seeds, and flaxseeds are excellent sources of essential fatty acids, including omega-3s and omega-6s, which help maintain the skin's lipid barrier and support hydration. They also provide vitamin E, an antioxidant that protects collagen fibers from oxidative stress and promotes skin elasticity. Enjoy a handful of nuts or seeds as a nutritious snack or add them to cereals, salads, or homemade granola for added collagen-boosting benefits.

The Role of Hydration in Skin Radiance

Achieving radiant, youthful skin involves more than just topical treatments—it begins with hydration from within. In "Beauty Unveiled: Collagen Supplements, Diet, and the Secret to Radiant Skin", we explore the vital role that hydration plays in maintaining skin health and enhancing your natural beauty.

Why Hydration Matters

Hydration is essential for skin health as it directly impacts the skin's appearance, texture, and overall radiance. The skin is the body's largest organ and serves as a barrier to protect against environmental aggressors, such as pollutants and UV rays. When adequately hydrated, the skin maintains its elasticity, suppleness, and ability to repair itself.

Impact of Dehydration on Skin

Insufficient hydration can lead to various skin issues, including dryness, flakiness, dullness, and accelerated signs of aging such as fine lines and wrinkles. When the skin lacks proper hydration, it may appear rough, uneven, and more prone to irritation and sensitivity. Additionally, dehydration can compromise the skin's natural barrier function, making it susceptible to infections and inflammation.

Hydration and Collagen Production

Hydration plays a crucial role in collagen production, which is essential for maintaining skin elasticity and firmness. Collagen is a structural protein that forms the framework of the skin, supporting its structure and preventing sagging. Adequate hydration ensures optimal circulation of nutrients and oxygen to skin cells, facilitating collagen synthesis and repair processes.

Optimal Hydration Tips for Radiant Skin

1. **Drink Plenty of Water:** Aim to drink at least 8 glasses (about 2 liters) of water per day to maintain hydration levels. Water helps flush out toxins from the body and keeps skin cells hydrated from within.

2. **Eat Water-Rich Foods:** Incorporate hydrating foods such as fruits (e.g., watermelon, oranges, and berries) and vegetables (e.g., cucumber, celery, and spinach) into your diet. These foods not only provide water but also essential vitamins, minerals, and antioxidants that support skin health.

3. **Use Hydrating Skincare Products:** Choose moisturizers and serums that contain hydrating ingredients such as hyaluronic acid, glycerin, and

ceramides. These ingredients help attract moisture to the skin and maintain hydration throughout the day.

4. **Limit Alcohol and Caffeine:** Alcohol and caffeine can dehydrate the body and, consequently, the skin. Moderation is key, and it's beneficial to balance their consumption with increased water intake.

5. **Protect Against External Factors:** Protect your skin from harsh environmental conditions such as dry air, wind, and sun exposure. Use sunscreen daily, wear protective clothing, and consider using a humidifier indoors to maintain optimal moisture levels in the air.

Hydration and Overall Well-Being

Beyond skin health, staying hydrated supports overall well-being, including digestion, circulation, and cognitive function. Proper hydration helps regulate body temperature, lubricates joints, and aids in the transportation of nutrients and oxygen throughout the body.

Collagen Supplements and Beauty

Enhancing Skin Elasticity and Firmness

Achieving and maintaining youthful, firm skin is a common goal for many individuals seeking to enhance their natural beauty. In "Beauty Unveiled: Collagen Supplements, Diet, and the Secret to Radiant Skin", we delve into effective strategies and practices to improve skin elasticity and firmness, key elements in maintaining a vibrant complexion.

Understanding Skin Elasticity and Firmness

Skin elasticity refers to the skin's ability to stretch and return to its original shape and firmness. Collagen and elastin fibers in the dermis provide structural support and resilience to the skin. As we age, collagen production naturally declines, resulting in a loss of skin elasticity and firmness. Factors such as sun exposure, smoking, dehydration, and poor nutrition can further accelerate this process, leading to sagging skin, wrinkles, and fine lines.

Effective Strategies to Enhance Skin Elasticity and Firmness

1. **Collagen Supplements:** Collagen supplements provide essential amino acids that support collagen synthesis and promote skin elasticity. Types I and III collagen, often derived from bovine or marine sources, are particularly beneficial for skin health. Regular intake of collagen supplements can help improve skin texture, reduce wrinkles, and enhance overall skin firmness.

2. **Healthy Diet:** A balanced diet rich in vitamins, minerals, antioxidants, and essential fatty acids is crucial for supporting skin elasticity and firmness. Include foods such as fruits, vegetables, lean proteins, nuts, seeds, and whole grains. These foods provide nutrients like vitamin C, vitamin E, zinc, and omega-3 fatty acids, which promote collagen production, protect against oxidative stress, and maintain skin hydration.

3. **Hydration:** Adequate hydration is essential for maintaining skin elasticity. Drink plenty of water throughout the day to keep skin cells hydrated and support optimal collagen synthesis. Hydrating skincare products containing ingredients like hyaluronic acid and glycerin can also help attract and retain moisture in the skin, enhancing elasticity and firmness.

4. **Sun Protection:** Protecting your skin from UV damage is crucial for preserving collagen and elastin fibers. Always apply sunscreen with broad-spectrum protection (SPF 30 or higher) before sun exposure, and wear protective clothing, hats, and sunglasses. Sunscreen helps prevent photoaging, reduces the breakdown of collagen, and maintains skin elasticity.

5. **Exercise and Movement:** Regular physical activity promotes blood circulation and delivery of oxygen and nutrients to the skin, supporting collagen production and skin firmness. Incorporate exercises that engage facial muscles, such as facial yoga or massage techniques, to improve muscle tone and skin elasticity.

6. **Skincare Routine:** Establish a skincare regimen tailored to your skin type and concerns. Use gentle cleansers, moisturizers, and serums containing ingredients like retinoids, peptides, and vitamin C to boost collagen production, improve skin texture, and enhance firmness. Avoid harsh products that can strip the skin of natural oils and contribute to dryness or irritation.

Lifestyle Considerations

- **Avoid Smoking:** Smoking accelerates collagen breakdown and impairs blood flow to the skin, leading to premature aging, wrinkles, and loss of elasticity. Quitting smoking can significantly improve skin health and firmness over time.

- **Manage Stress:** Chronic stress can contribute to skin aging by triggering inflammation and hormonal imbalances. Practice stress management techniques such as meditation, yoga, deep breathing exercises, or hobbies to promote relaxation and support skin elasticity.

Combatting Signs of Aging with Collagen

As we age, our skin undergoes natural changes that can manifest as wrinkles, fine lines, sagging, and loss of elasticity. In "Beauty Unveiled: Collagen Supplements, Diet, and the Secret to Radiant Skin", we explore how collagen supplementation can effectively combat these signs of aging, helping you maintain a youthful and radiant complexion.

Understanding Aging Skin

The aging process affects the skin in several ways:

1. **Collagen Depletion:** Collagen is a protein that provides structural support to the skin. With age, collagen production decreases, leading to a loss of skin firmness, elasticity, and resilience.
2. **Elastin Breakdown:** Elastin fibers, which contribute to skin elasticity, also diminish over time. This contributes to the formation of wrinkles and sagging skin.
3. **Decreased Hydration:** Aging skin tends to become drier as the skin's ability to retain moisture decreases. This can exacerbate the appearance of fine lines and wrinkles.

4. **Environmental Damage:** Factors such as UV exposure, pollution, and lifestyle habits (e.g., smoking, poor diet) can accelerate skin aging by causing oxidative stress and collagen degradation.

How Collagen Supplements Help Combat Signs of Aging

Collagen supplements, particularly those containing hydrolyzed collagen peptides, offer a potent solution to support skin health and combat visible signs of aging:

1. **Boosting Collagen Production:** Collagen supplements provide amino acids such as glycine, proline, and hydroxyproline, which are essential for collagen synthesis. By replenishing these building blocks, collagen supplements help stimulate the body's natural production of collagen, promoting firmer, smoother skin and reducing the appearance of wrinkles.

2. **Improving Skin Elasticity:** Collagen peptides derived from sources like bovine or marine collagen are easily absorbed by the body. They support the skin's elasticity by enhancing dermal collagen density and improving skin hydration levels. This results in skin that feels more supple and resilient.

3. **Reducing Wrinkle Depth:** Clinical studies have demonstrated that regular supplementation with collagen peptides can lead to a significant reduction in wrinkle depth and overall improvement in skin texture. These peptides work to restore the skin's structural integrity, smoothing out fine lines and wrinkles over time.

4. **Enhancing Skin Hydration:** Collagen supplements not only promote collagen synthesis but also help retain moisture in the skin. This dual action supports optimal hydration levels, improving skin plumpness and radiance.

5. **Supporting Overall Skin Health:** Beyond aesthetic benefits, collagen supplementation supports skin health by protecting against UV-induced damage, reducing inflammation, and promoting faster wound healing. This comprehensive approach helps maintain skin integrity and resilience against environmental stressors.

Incorporating Collagen into Your Routine

To maximize the anti-aging benefits of collagen supplementation:

- **Choose Quality Supplements:** Opt for collagen supplements from reputable brands that prioritize quality and purity. Look for products that are hydrolyzed for better absorption and free from unnecessary additives or allergens.

- **Follow Recommended Dosage:** Consult with a healthcare provider or dermatologist to determine the appropriate dosage of collagen supplements based on your individual needs and health goals.

- **Combine with a Healthy Lifestyle:** Support collagen synthesis by maintaining a balanced diet rich in vitamins, minerals, and antioxidants. Stay hydrated, protect your skin from sun exposure, and adopt a skincare routine that includes products aimed at promoting collagen production and skin hydration.

Clinical Studies and Evidence

In the realm of skincare and beauty, understanding the scientific evidence behind treatments and supplements is crucial. "Beauty Unveiled: Collagen Supplements, Diet, and the Secret to Radiant Skin" explores the clinical studies and evidence supporting the effectiveness of collagen supplements in promoting skin health and enhancing radiance.

The Role of Collagen in Skin Health

Collagen is a fundamental protein in the skin that provides structure, elasticity, and strength. As we age, natural collagen production declines, leading to visible signs of aging such as wrinkles, fine lines, and sagging skin. Collagen supplements aim to replenish and support the body's collagen stores, thereby improving skin elasticity, hydration, and overall appearance.

Key Findings from Clinical Studies

1. **Improvement in Skin Elasticity:** Several clinical studies have demonstrated that collagen supplementation can significantly enhance skin elasticity. For example, a study published in the Journal of Cosmetic Dermatology found that participants who

took collagen peptides experienced improvements in skin elasticity and moisture content compared to a placebo group.

2. **Reduction in Wrinkle Depth and Appearance:** Research has shown that collagen peptides can reduce the depth of wrinkles and improve overall skin texture. A study published in Skin Pharmacology and Physiology reported that daily oral supplementation with collagen peptides led to a visible reduction in eye wrinkle volume after just eight weeks of use.

3. **Hydration and Moisture Retention:** Collagen supplements have been shown to support skin hydration by increasing the skin's ability to retain moisture. Studies indicate that collagen peptides help enhance the skin's natural barrier function, preventing water loss and maintaining optimal hydration levels.

4. **Collagen Synthesis Support:** Clinical evidence suggests that collagen supplementation stimulates the body's own collagen synthesis processes. This includes providing essential amino acids like glycine, proline, and hydroxyproline, which are necessary for collagen production in the skin.

5. **Overall Skin Health Benefits:** Beyond aesthetic improvements, collagen supplementation has been

associated with broader skin health benefits. These include protection against UV-induced damage, reduction in inflammation, and support for wound healing processes.

Quality and Considerations

When evaluating the effectiveness of collagen supplements, it's essential to consider the quality of clinical studies:

- **Study Design:** Look for randomized, placebo-controlled trials with a sufficient number of participants and clear endpoints related to skin health outcomes.
- **Publication in Peer-Reviewed Journals:** Studies published in reputable scientific journals undergo rigorous peer review to ensure methodological soundness and validity of findings.
- **Consistency of Results:** Reliable clinical evidence often includes multiple studies showing consistent results across diverse populations and settings.

Practical Application and Recommendations

Based on current clinical evidence, incorporating collagen supplements into your skincare regimen can contribute to healthier, more radiant skin. When selecting collagen products, opt for those that are hydrolyzed for better absorption and sourced from reputable manufacturers. It's also beneficial to consult with a healthcare provider or dermatologist to determine the appropriate dosage and assess potential interactions with other supplements or medications.

Integrating Collagen into Your Beauty Routine

DIY Collagen Masks and Treatments

In your journey towards radiant and youthful skin, incorporating DIY collagen masks and treatments can complement your skincare routine effectively. "Beauty Unveiled: Collagen Supplements, Diet, and the Secret to Radiant Skin" explores simple yet powerful ways to harness the benefits of collagen through homemade treatments that nourish and rejuvenate your skin.

Understanding Collagen and Skin Health

Collagen is a vital protein that maintains skin elasticity, firmness, and hydration. As we age, collagen production naturally declines, leading to visible signs of aging such as wrinkles, fine lines, and sagging skin. DIY collagen masks and treatments offer a natural approach to stimulate collagen synthesis, improve skin texture, and enhance overall radiance.

Benefits of DIY Collagen Masks

1. **Enhanced Skin Hydration:** DIY masks can help replenish moisture levels in the skin, promoting a plump and supple complexion. Ingredients such as honey, yogurt, and avocado provide hydration while supporting collagen production.

2. **Improved Elasticity:** Collagen masks enriched with natural ingredients like egg whites or aloe vera can help tighten and firm the skin, reducing the appearance of fine lines and promoting a more youthful appearance.

3. **Reduced Fine Lines and Wrinkles:** DIY treatments containing collagen-boosting ingredients such as vitamin C-rich fruits (e.g., strawberries, oranges) or green tea can help diminish the depth and visibility of wrinkles over time.

4. **Glowing Complexion:** Regular use of DIY collagen masks can impart a radiant glow to the skin by improving circulation, removing impurities, and enhancing overall skin tone.

DIY Collagen Mask Recipes

Here are a few simple and effective DIY collagen mask recipes to try at home:

1. Hydrating Yogurt and Honey Mask:

- Ingredients:
    - 1 tablespoon plain yogurt
    - 1 tablespoon honey
    - 1 teaspoon lemon juice (optional)
- Instructions:
    1. Mix the yogurt and honey together until smooth.
    2. Add lemon juice if desired for added brightening effect.
    3. Apply a thick layer to clean skin and leave on for 15-20 minutes.
    4. Rinse off with lukewarm water and pat dry. Follow with moisturizer.

2. Nourishing Avocado and Egg White Mask:

- Ingredients:
    - 1/2 ripe avocado, mashed
    - 1 egg white
    - 1 teaspoon olive oil

- Instructions:

    1. Combine mashed avocado, egg white, and olive oil in a bowl until well blended.

    2. Apply the mixture evenly to your face and neck.

    3. Leave on for 15-20 minutes or until dry.

    4. Rinse off with cool water and gently pat dry. Follow with your regular skincare routine.

3. Brightening Strawberry and Green Tea Mask:

- Ingredients:

    o 2-3 ripe strawberries, mashed

    o 1 tablespoon brewed green tea (cooled)

    o 1 tablespoon plain yogurt

- Instructions:

    1. Mash the strawberries and mix with brewed green tea and yogurt.

    2. Apply the mixture to clean skin, focusing on areas prone to pigmentation or dullness.

    3. Leave on for 15-20 minutes.

    4. Rinse off with lukewarm water and pat dry. Follow with moisturizer.

Tips for DIY Collagen Treatments

- **Consistency is Key:** Incorporate DIY collagen masks into your skincare routine 1-2 times per week for best results.
- **Patch Test:** Before applying any new ingredients to your face, perform a patch test on a small area of skin to check for any allergic reactions or sensitivities.
- **Fresh Ingredients:** Use fresh, high-quality ingredients to maximize the potency and benefits of your DIY collagen treatments.

Best Practices for Incorporating Collagen Supplements

In the pursuit of radiant and youthful skin, incorporating collagen supplements into your daily routine can significantly enhance skin health and appearance. "Beauty Unveiled: Collagen Supplements, Diet, and the Secret to Radiant Skin" outlines the best practices for effectively integrating collagen supplements to optimize their benefits and achieve a glowing complexion.

Understanding Collagen Supplements

Collagen supplements are derived from sources such as bovine (cow), marine (fish), or poultry (chicken) collagen. They typically come in the form of capsules, tablets, powders, or liquid formulations. These supplements aim to replenish collagen levels in the body, supporting skin elasticity, hydration, and overall skin health.

Best Practices for Incorporating Collagen Supplements

1. **Choose High-Quality Supplements:** Opt for collagen supplements from reputable brands known for their quality and purity. Look for products that are

hydrolyzed, as this form ensures better absorption and bioavailability.

2. **Consult with a Healthcare Professional:** Before starting any new supplement regimen, especially if you have underlying health conditions or are pregnant/nursing, consult with a healthcare provider or dermatologist. They can provide personalized recommendations based on your individual needs.

3. **Follow Recommended Dosage:** Adhere to the recommended dosage as indicated on the supplement packaging or as advised by your healthcare provider. Consistency is key to experiencing the full benefits of collagen supplementation.

4. **Consider Timing and Method of Consumption:**
   o **Timing:** Collagen supplements can typically be taken at any time of the day, with or without food. Choose a time that aligns with your schedule and allows for consistent daily intake.
   o **Method:** Collagen supplements are available in various forms. Powders can be easily mixed into beverages or smoothies, while capsules or tablets are convenient for those on the go. Select a form that fits your lifestyle and preferences.

5. **Combine with a Balanced Diet:** While collagen supplements provide essential amino acids for collagen synthesis, supporting your skin with a balanced diet rich in vitamins, minerals, and antioxidants further enhances their efficacy. Incorporate collagen-boosting foods such as fruits, vegetables, lean proteins, and healthy fats into your meals.

6. **Stay Hydrated:** Adequate hydration is crucial for skin health and collagen synthesis. Drink plenty of water throughout the day to keep your skin hydrated from within and optimize the benefits of collagen supplements.

7. **Monitor Results:** Pay attention to how your skin responds to collagen supplementation over time. Notice any improvements in skin elasticity, hydration, and overall radiance. Adjust your regimen as needed based on your observations and feedback from your healthcare provider.

Additional Considerations:

- **Consistency:** Incorporating collagen supplements into your daily routine consistently is essential for achieving and maintaining optimal results.

- **Patience:** While some individuals may notice improvements in skin texture and appearance relatively quickly, it may take several weeks to months for significant changes to become noticeable. Be patient and persistent with your regimen.
- **Pair with Skincare Routine:** Complement your collagen supplementation with a tailored skincare routine that includes cleansers, moisturizers, and serums aimed at promoting collagen production and maintaining skin health.

Complementary Skincare Practices

Achieving radiant, youthful skin goes beyond just using collagen supplements—it involves adopting a holistic approach to skincare. In "Beauty Unveiled: Collagen Supplements, Diet, and the Secret to Radiant Skin", we explore essential complementary skincare practices that enhance the benefits of collagen supplementation and promote overall skin health.

1. Cleansing Routine

A proper cleansing routine forms the foundation of a healthy skincare regimen. Cleansing removes impurities, excess oil, and makeup residue that can clog pores and contribute to skin dullness. Choose a gentle cleanser suited to your skin type (dry, oily, combination) and cleanse your face twice daily—morning and night—to maintain clean and fresh skin.

2. Exfoliation

Regular exfoliation helps slough off dead skin cells, promoting cell turnover and revealing smoother, brighter skin underneath. Use a gentle exfoliating scrub or chemical exfoliant (e.g., AHAs or BHAs) 1-2 times per week to prevent dullness, improve skin texture, and allow better absorption of skincare products, including collagen supplements.

3. Moisturizing

Hydration is essential for maintaining skin elasticity and suppleness. Choose a moisturizer that suits your skin type and contains hydrating ingredients like hyaluronic acid, glycerin, or ceramides. Apply moisturizer daily after cleansing to lock in moisture and create a protective barrier against environmental stressors.

4. Sun Protection

Protecting your skin from UV damage is crucial for preventing premature aging and maintaining collagen levels. Apply a broad-spectrum sunscreen with SPF 30 or higher every morning, even on cloudy days or during winter months. Reapply sunscreen every 2 hours when outdoors or after swimming or sweating.

5. Anti-Aging Serums

Incorporate anti-aging serums into your skincare routine to target specific concerns such as fine lines, wrinkles, and loss of elasticity. Look for serums containing ingredients like vitamin C, retinoids, peptides, or growth factors, which promote collagen production, improve skin texture, and enhance overall skin tone.

6. Facial Massage and Exercises

Facial massages and exercises can help stimulate blood circulation, relax facial muscles, and promote lymphatic drainage. Incorporate gentle massage techniques or facial yoga into your routine to boost circulation, reduce puffiness, and enhance the absorption of skincare products.

7. Healthy Lifestyle Habits

Support your skincare regimen with healthy lifestyle habits that promote overall well-being and skin health:

- **Nutritious Diet:** Consume a balanced diet rich in fruits, vegetables, lean proteins, and healthy fats to provide essential nutrients for skin health and collagen synthesis.
- **Hydration:** Drink plenty of water throughout the day to keep your skin hydrated and support optimal collagen production.
- **Quality Sleep:** Aim for 7-9 hours of quality sleep each night to allow your skin to repair and regenerate.
- **Stress Management:** Practice stress-reducing activities such as yoga, meditation, or deep breathing exercises to minimize stress-induced skin issues.

8. Regular Skin Check-Ups

Schedule regular visits with a dermatologist or skincare professional for skin assessments and personalized recommendations. They can help identify skin concerns early, provide targeted treatments, and adjust your skincare regimen as needed to achieve and maintain healthy, radiant skin.

The Link Between Diet, Lifestyle, and Skin Appearance

Impact of Diet on Skin Conditions

The old adage "you are what you eat" holds true when it comes to skincare. In "Beauty Unveiled: Collagen Supplements, Diet, and the Secret to Radiant Skin", we explore the profound impact that diet has on various skin conditions and overall skin health. Understanding how dietary choices influence skin can empower you to make informed decisions that promote a clear, radiant complexion.

Nutrients Essential for Healthy Skin

1. **Antioxidants:** Found in fruits, vegetables, and nuts, antioxidants like vitamins A, C, and E help protect skin cells from oxidative stress caused by free radicals. They contribute to skin repair, reduce inflammation, and support collagen production.

2. **Omega-3 Fatty Acids:** Found in fatty fish (salmon, mackerel), flaxseeds, and walnuts, omega-3s help

maintain skin hydration, reduce inflammation, and support overall skin barrier function.

3. **Vitamins and Minerals:** Zinc, selenium, and vitamin D are crucial for skin health. Zinc aids in wound healing and controls oil production, while selenium protects against sun damage. Vitamin D supports skin cell growth, repair, and metabolism.

4. **Proteins:** Essential for collagen and elastin synthesis, proteins from sources like lean meats, poultry, dairy, and legumes help maintain skin structure and elasticity.

Impact of Specific Foods on Skin Conditions

1. **Acne:** High glycemic index foods (sugar, refined carbohydrates) can exacerbate acne by increasing insulin levels and inflammation. Incorporating low glycemic index foods (whole grains, fruits, vegetables) and foods rich in zinc and antioxidants (nuts, seeds, leafy greens) may help manage acne.

2. **Eczema and Dermatitis:** Foods that trigger inflammation (dairy, gluten, processed foods) may worsen symptoms. Anti-inflammatory foods (fatty fish, berries, turmeric) and probiotic-rich foods (yogurt, kefir) can support skin barrier function and reduce flare-ups.

3. **Dry Skin:** Hydration is key for combating dry skin. Drinking plenty of water and consuming water-rich fruits and vegetables (cucumbers, watermelon) help maintain skin moisture levels. Omega-3 fatty acids from fish and plant sources also support skin hydration.

Healthy Eating Habits for Radiant Skin

1. **Hydration:** Drink at least 8 glasses of water daily to maintain skin hydration and flush out toxins. Herbal teas and infused water are excellent hydrating alternatives.

2. **Balanced Diet:** Incorporate a variety of nutrient-dense foods into your meals, including colorful fruits and vegetables, lean proteins, whole grains, and healthy fats. Aim for a rainbow of colors on your plate to ensure a diverse intake of vitamins and antioxidants.

3. **Limit Sugar and Processed Foods:** Excess sugar and processed foods can contribute to inflammation and premature aging of the skin. Opt for natural sweeteners like honey or maple syrup and choose whole, unprocessed foods whenever possible.

4. **Moderate Alcohol and Caffeine:** Both alcohol and caffeine can dehydrate the skin. Consume these

beverages in moderation and balance them with hydrating options like water or herbal tea.

Lifestyle Habits for Healthy, Glowing Skin

Achieving radiant and healthy skin is not just about skincare products and supplements; it also involves adopting beneficial lifestyle habits. In "Beauty Unveiled: Collagen Supplements, Diet, and the Secret to Radiant Skin", we explore key lifestyle practices that can enhance the health and appearance of your skin, promoting a natural glow from within.

1. Prioritize Sleep

Quality sleep is crucial for skin health and overall well-being. During sleep, the body repairs and regenerates skin cells, promotes collagen production, and balances hormone levels. Aim for 7-9 hours of uninterrupted sleep each night to support skin renewal and maintain a youthful complexion.

2. Manage Stress Effectively

Chronic stress can trigger skin issues such as acne, eczema, and premature aging. Practice stress management techniques such as meditation, deep breathing exercises, yoga, or hobbies that promote relaxation. Managing stress helps reduce cortisol levels, inflammation, and oxidative stress, which can contribute to skin dullness and breakouts.

3. Exercise Regularly

Regular physical activity improves blood circulation, delivering oxygen and nutrients to skin cells and promoting detoxification. Exercise also helps reduce stress and supports hormone balance, contributing to clearer, healthier-looking skin. Aim for at least 30 minutes of moderate exercise most days of the week for optimal skin benefits.

4. Protect from Sun Exposure

UV rays from the sun accelerate skin aging, causing wrinkles, dark spots, and loss of elasticity. Protect your skin by wearing broad-spectrum sunscreen with SPF 30 or higher every day, even on cloudy days or during winter. Reapply sunscreen every 2 hours when outdoors and wear protective clothing, hats, and sunglasses to shield your skin from UV damage.

5. Avoid Smoking and Limit Alcohol Consumption

Smoking accelerates skin aging by damaging collagen and elastin fibers, leading to wrinkles and sagging skin. Quitting smoking or avoiding exposure to secondhand smoke can help preserve skin elasticity and promote a more youthful appearance. Limit alcohol consumption, as excessive alcohol intake can dehydrate the skin and impair its natural barrier function.

6. Maintain Hydration

Proper hydration is essential for skin health and radiance. Drink plenty of water throughout the day to keep your skin hydrated and flush out toxins. Herbal teas, infused water, and hydrating foods like fruits and vegetables also contribute to overall hydration levels and support skin elasticity.

7. Follow a Consistent Skincare Routine

Establishing a daily skincare regimen tailored to your skin type and concerns is essential for maintaining healthy skin. Cleanse your face twice daily, exfoliate regularly to remove dead skin cells, moisturize to lock in hydration, and use serums or treatments to address specific skin issues. Choose skincare products formulated with gentle, effective ingredients that support skin barrier function and promote a balanced complexion.

8. Get Regular Skin Check-Ups

Schedule regular visits with a dermatologist or skincare professional for skin assessments and personalized recommendations. Early detection of skin concerns allows for timely treatment and management, ensuring your skin remains healthy and radiant.

Stress Management and Its Effect on Skin

In the pursuit of radiant and healthy skin, stress management plays a pivotal role. "Beauty Unveiled: Collagen Supplements, Diet, and the Secret to Radiant Skin" delves into the profound impact of stress on skin health and explores effective strategies for managing stress to promote a clear, youthful complexion.

Understanding the Stress-Skin Connection

Stress is a natural physiological response triggered by various factors such as work pressure, personal relationships, financial concerns, or health issues. When stress becomes chronic or overwhelming, it can manifest in physical symptoms, including skin problems. The connection between stress and skin health is bidirectional, meaning stress can exacerbate existing skin conditions and vice versa.

Effects of Stress on the Skin

1. **Acne and Breakouts:** Stress triggers the release of hormones like cortisol and adrenaline, which increase oil production in the skin. Excess oil can clog pores and lead to acne breakouts, particularly in individuals prone to oily or combination skin types.

2. **Accelerated Aging:** Chronic stress accelerates the aging process by promoting the breakdown of collagen and elastin fibers in the skin. This can result in the formation of wrinkles, fine lines, and sagging skin, making the skin appear dull and less elastic.

3. **Skin Sensitivity and Irritation:** Stress weakens the skin's natural barrier function, making it more susceptible to environmental irritants, allergens, and inflammatory responses. This can exacerbate conditions like eczema, psoriasis, and rosacea, causing redness, itching, and flares.

4. **Impaired Skin Healing:** Stress interferes with the skin's ability to repair and regenerate. Wounds, cuts, or blemishes may take longer to heal, and the skin's overall

resilience and ability to recover from damage are compromised.

Effective Stress Management Strategies

1. **Mindfulness and Relaxation Techniques:** Practice mindfulness meditation, deep breathing exercises, progressive muscle relaxation, or yoga to promote relaxation and reduce stress levels. These techniques help calm the mind, lower cortisol levels, and improve overall well-being.

2. **Regular Exercise:** Engage in regular physical activity such as walking, jogging, dancing, or yoga to release endorphins (feel-good hormones) and alleviate stress. Exercise improves blood circulation, delivers oxygen and nutrients to the skin, and supports overall skin health.

3. **Healthy Lifestyle Choices:** Maintain a balanced diet rich in fruits, vegetables, lean proteins, and whole grains. Avoid excessive consumption of caffeine, alcohol, and sugary foods, which can exacerbate stress and negatively impact skin health.

4. **Quality Sleep:** Prioritize adequate sleep of 7-9 hours per night to allow the body and skin to repair and regenerate. Establish a bedtime routine, create a

relaxing sleep environment, and avoid screen time before bed to promote restful sleep.

5. **Social Support:** Build and nurture strong social connections with friends, family, or support groups. Sharing concerns and experiences with others can provide emotional support and reduce feelings of stress and anxiety.

6. **Professional Help:** Seek guidance from a therapist, counselor, or healthcare provider if stress becomes overwhelming or affects daily life significantly. They can offer personalized strategies and support to manage stress effectively.

Beauty from Within: Real-life Success Stories

Testimonials and Case Studies

Discover how individuals have transformed their skin health with the guidance and principles outlined in "Beauty Unveiled: Collagen Supplements, Diet, and the Secret to Radiant Skin". These testimonials and case studies offer firsthand accounts of the transformative effects of collagen supplements and holistic skincare practices on achieving radiant, youthful skin.

1. Emily's Radiant Transformation

"For years, I struggled with dull, uneven skin and premature signs of aging. Determined to find a solution, I turned to 'Beauty Unveiled' and incorporated collagen supplements into my daily routine. With the guidance on diet, skincare practices, and stress management, I've seen remarkable improvements. My skin feels firmer, smoother, and has a natural glow that I haven't seen in years. I'm thrilled with the results!"

2. James' Journey to Clear Skin

"As someone who battled persistent acne, I was skeptical about trying new skincare approaches. However, after reading 'Beauty Unveiled' and understanding the impact of diet and supplements on skin health, I decided to give it a try. By integrating collagen supplements and adopting healthier eating habits, my breakouts have significantly reduced, and my skin looks clearer and more balanced. This book has been a game-changer for me!"

3. Sarah's Age-Defying Success

"Approaching my forties, I noticed fine lines and loss of elasticity creeping in. 'Beauty Unveiled' provided me with valuable insights into the role of collagen in combating signs of aging. With consistent use of collagen supplements and following the recommended skincare routines, my skin feels firmer, and those fine lines have visibly diminished. I'm thrilled to have found a natural way to maintain youthful-looking skin!"

4. John's Stress Relief and Skin Improvement

"Stress was taking a toll on my skin, causing flare-ups and sensitivity. 'Beauty Unveiled' taught me the importance of stress management and its impact on skin health. By

incorporating mindfulness practices and nutritional changes, along with collagen supplements, I've noticed a significant reduction in redness and irritation. My skin feels more resilient, and I finally feel in control of my skin's health."

5. Lisa's Holistic Skincare Journey

"Struggling with eczema and dry, sensitive skin, I turned to 'Beauty Unveiled' for holistic solutions. By following the advice on nutrition, hydration, and skincare routines, including DIY collagen masks, my skin has undergone a remarkable transformation. The eczema flare-ups are less frequent, and my skin feels nourished and more comfortable than ever. This book has been a lifeline for me!"

Conclusion

These testimonials and case studies highlight the diverse ways individuals have benefited from the principles shared in "Beauty Unveiled: Collagen Supplements, Diet, and the Secret to Radiant Skin". Whether combating signs of aging, managing skin conditions, or enhancing overall skin health, these stories demonstrate the power of collagen supplements and holistic skincare practices in achieving radiant and healthy skin. Explore the transformative possibilities for yourself and embark on your journey to glowing skin with confidence and knowledge from book "Beauty Unveiled".

Personal Journeys to Radiant Skin

In "Beauty Unveiled: Collagen Supplements, Diet, and the Secret to Radiant Skin", we celebrate personal stories of individuals who have embarked on transformative journeys to achieve radiant and healthy skin. These inspiring narratives showcase the power of collagen supplements, dietary adjustments, and holistic skincare practices in revitalizing their skin and boosting their confidence.

1. Emma's Renewed Confidence

"Struggling with dry, lackluster skin for years, I felt self-conscious and frustrated. 'Beauty Unveiled' introduced me to the benefits of collagen supplements and the impact of diet on skin health. By incorporating collagen into my daily routine and adopting a diet rich in antioxidants and omega-3s, my skin began to transform. It became more hydrated, smoother, and had a natural radiance I hadn't seen in ages. This journey has not only improved my skin but also boosted my confidence!"

2. Michael's Journey to Clearer Complexion

"Dealing with persistent acne into my twenties was disheartening. 'Beauty Unveiled' opened my eyes to the connection between diet, stress, and skin health. I started taking collagen supplements and made changes to my diet, reducing processed foods and incorporating more whole foods. Gradually, my breakouts diminished, and my skin tone evened out. Today, my skin looks clearer and feels healthier than ever. This journey has been empowering and transformative."

3. Sarah's Anti-Aging Success

"Approaching my thirties, I began noticing fine lines and dullness in my complexion. 'Beauty Unveiled' inspired me to take proactive steps in preserving my skin's youthfulness. I started using collagen supplements daily and adjusted my skincare routine to focus on hydration and anti-aging ingredients. Over time, I've noticed a significant improvement in skin elasticity, reduced fine lines, and a brighter complexion. This journey has taught me the importance of nourishing my skin from within."

4. David's Stress-Free Skincare Routine

"Managing a high-stress job took a toll on my skin, causing frequent breakouts and sensitivity. 'Beauty Unveiled' guided me toward stress management techniques and the role of collagen in skin repair. By incorporating mindfulness practices, regular exercise, and collagen supplements, I've seen a remarkable reduction in breakouts and redness. My skin feels more resilient, and I've regained control over my skin's health. This journey has been transformative for both my skin and overall well-being."

5. Olivia's Holistic Skincare Journey

"Living with eczema was challenging, and I struggled to find effective solutions. 'Beauty Unveiled' introduced me to holistic skincare practices, including dietary adjustments and DIY collagen masks. By eliminating triggers from my diet and nourishing my skin with collagen-rich treatments, my eczema flare-ups have reduced significantly. My skin feels calmer, more hydrated, and I've regained my confidence. This journey has shown me the power of embracing a holistic approach to skincare."

Conclusion

These personal journeys exemplify the transformative impact of collagen supplements, dietary modifications, and holistic skincare practices detailed in "Beauty Unveiled: Collagen Supplements, Diet, and the Secret to Radiant Skin". By sharing these stories, we celebrate the resilience and commitment of individuals who have achieved radiant, healthy skin through dedication and knowledge. Explore their journeys, be inspired, and embark on your own path to glowing skin with confidence and determination.

Appendix

Glossary of Key Terms

Explore the essential terms and concepts related to skincare, collagen supplements, and diet featured in "Beauty Unveiled: Collagen Supplements, Diet, and the Secret to Radiant Skin". This glossary provides clarity and understanding to help you navigate the journey to achieving radiant and healthy skin.

1. **Collagen:** A protein that provides structure to the skin, promoting elasticity and firmness.

2. **Collagen Peptides:** Hydrolyzed collagen broken down into smaller molecules for easier absorption by the body.

3. **Antioxidants:** Compounds that protect skin cells from damage caused by free radicals, which can accelerate aging and cause skin disorders.

4. **Hyaluronic Acid:** A substance naturally found in the skin that attracts and retains moisture, promoting hydration and plumpness.

5. **Elastin:** A protein similar to collagen that gives skin its elasticity and resilience.

6. **Free Radicals:** Unstable molecules that can damage skin cells and accelerate aging through oxidative stress.

7. **Glycation:** The process by which sugar molecules attach to proteins like collagen, causing them to become stiff and prone to damage, contributing to aging.

8. **Omega-3 Fatty Acids:** Essential fatty acids found in fish, nuts, and seeds that support skin health, hydration, and inflammation reduction.

9. **Vitamin C:** An antioxidant that helps repair and regenerate tissues, promotes collagen production, and protects against UV damage.

10. **Retinoids:** Vitamin A derivatives that promote cell turnover, reduce wrinkles, and improve skin texture and tone.

11. **SPF:** Sun Protection Factor, a measure of how well sunscreen protects against UVB rays that cause sunburn and skin cancer.

12. **Exfoliation:** The process of removing dead skin cells from the skin's surface to reveal smoother, brighter skin.

13. **Hydration:** The process of adding moisture to the skin to maintain its elasticity, plumpness, and overall health.

14. **Probiotics:** Beneficial bacteria that support gut health and may improve skin conditions by reducing inflammation and supporting the skin barrier.

15. **Essential Nutrients:** Vitamins, minerals, and other compounds necessary for healthy skin function, repair, and regeneration.

16. **Stress Management:** Techniques and practices that reduce stress levels, which can improve skin conditions and overall well-being.

17. **Skincare Routine:** A personalized regimen of cleansing, exfoliating, moisturizing, and treating the skin to maintain its health and appearance.

18. **Dermatologist:** A medical doctor specializing in diagnosing and treating skin disorders and conditions.

19. **Holistic Approach:** Addressing skincare from a comprehensive perspective that considers internal factors (diet, stress, hydration) as well as external factors (products, treatments).

20. **DIY Masks:** Homemade skincare treatments using natural ingredients to nourish, hydrate, and treat the skin.

Understanding these key terms will empower you to make informed decisions about your skincare regimen. Enhance your skincare journey with knowledge and confidence, and unlock the secrets to achieving radiant and healthy skin naturally.

Additional Resources and References

"Beauty Unveiled: Collagen Supplements, Diet, and the Secret to Radiant Skin" provides a comprehensive guide to achieving healthy, glowing skin through collagen supplements, diet adjustments, and holistic skincare practices. Explore these additional resources and references to further enhance your understanding and journey towards radiant skin:

Books:

1. "The Wrinkle Cure" by Nicholas Perricone
2. "The Beauty of Dirty Skin" by Whitney Bowe, MD
3. "The Skincare Bible: Your No-Nonsense Guide to Great Skin" by Anjali Mahto, MD

Websites:

1. American Academy of Dermatology (AAD) - Skin Health Information: https://www.aad.org
2. National Institute of Health (NIH) - Dietary Supplements Fact Sheets: https://ods.od.nih.gov/factsheets/list-all/

Articles and Research Papers:

1. "Collagen: A Review on its Sources and Potential Cosmetic Applications" - Journal of Cosmetic Dermatology
2. "The Role of Nutrition for Skin Health: A Comprehensive Review" - International Journal of Molecular Sciences

Podcasts:

1. "The Beauty Brains" - Science-based skincare discussions
2. "The Healthy Skin Show" - Insights into skincare and skin health

Social Media Influencers:

Follow skincare experts and influencers who share valuable tips and insights on Instagram, YouTube, and TikTok.

Professional Organizations:

1. International Society of Dermatology (ISD)
2. Society of Cosmetic Chemists (SCC)

These resources and references will further enrich your knowledge and support your journey to achieving radiant and healthy skin as outlined in "Beauty Unveiled: Collagen Supplements, Diet, and the Secret to Radiant Skin". Stay informed, explore diverse perspectives, and continue to prioritize your skin's health and beauty with confidence and knowledge.